CW01239357

www.SportsHypnosis.co.uk

How to *Trick* a FAT Kid into Weight Loss

for Kids who Hate Diets & Exercise!

Stephen T Mycoe BA(Hons)

Copyright © 2012 Stephen Mycoe

All rights reserved. Please see page 105-106 for full Copyright & Disclaimer details.

ISBN: **1475249160**
ISBN-13: **978-1475249163**

Table of Contents

Introduction 1

Chapter One - The Reality of Obesity in Kids 9

    Diabetes in Kids..10

    Heart Disease in Children...12

    Hypertension in Children 13

    Thyroid Damage in Kids 14

    Sleep Apnoea in Overweight Kids 15

    Social Aspects of Child Obesity 16

    Cancer 17

Chapter Two - Weight Loss for Kids 19

    Body Fat and Calories in Children 21

    How to Tell if a Kid is Overweight 24

    A Balanced Diet for Kids...25

    The Five Main Food groups..27

    Kids and Meal Times 30

    Breakfast 33

    Lunch...40

Dinner / Evening Meal 43

Weight Loss and the Household Environment.............45

Protein Snacks for Kids...47

High Energy Foods and Drinks for Kids 51

Chapter Three - How to Trick a Kid into Weight Loss 55

Don't Pressurise Your Kids 55

Distraction and Taste Sensation 57

Educating your Kids to Cook. 61

Changing the Language you use. 63

Substituting the worst offenders. 64

Rewind the Corporate Brainwashing 65

Join in!...67

Chapter Four - How to Trick a Kid into Feeling Great! 69

Benefits of Exercise..70

How much Exercise? 72

How a Childs body responds to exercise......................74

Understanding exercise intensity 75

Getting involved...77

Chapter Five - How to Trick a Kid into Exercise! 79

   Activities that a Tricked Kid will Love...........................80

Chapter Six - House Hold Activities and Lifestyle changes that 'Trick' a Kid into burning Calories. 97

References 103

Copyright and Disclaimer 106

About Steve...108

ACKNOWLEDGMENTS

Thanks to Carolynne for her usual editorial enhancements including the all important sentence she added! The next book is 'in the post'! : 0

Introduction

The World is getting Fatter and it's beginning during Childhood!

Over Two Hundred Million Kids are overweight in the World and there is no indication that this trend is going to decline.

One problem is that parents of overweight kids are blissfully unaware of the problem*1. Parents are becoming so used to seeing fat kids that Fifty Seven Percent (57%) of Fathers and Thirty Three Percent (33%) of Mothers don't recognize obesity in their own children! This brings up several issues. *One;* overweight kids can't be supported and helped by their parents if they simply don't recognize the problem. *Two;* If parents perceptions are failing to identify overweight kids what other strategy can we instigate to help detect high body fat percentages in kids before they become clinically obese? We'll discover the answers to these question in subsequent chapters.

'…57% OF FATHERS AND 33% OF MOTHERS DON'T RECOGNISE OBESITY IN THEIR OWN KIDS!'

Even when we consider the parents who do recognize obesity in their kids, difficulties remain in getting an older child to eat well and exercise when they have already formed the behaviours and Psychological associations with a poor diet.

Overweight kids hate exercise, they are often no good at it, they are teased at school, they feel embarrassed getting involved in conventional sports and fear failure.

In addition there are mental health issues associated with kids being overweight. An overweight Child is vastly more likely to become depressed than a healthy Child *2.

These are just a few of the reasons why we need to 'trick' kids into adopting a healthy lifestyle whilst having fun - without them being aware of it!

It is essential to 'get them when they are young' in order to make sure kids are healthy in adulthood. If a child is unhealthy the likelihood that they will lead a healthy lifestyle when older and free of health issues is vastly reduced. This is even more worrying when you take into account the fact that the average adult who is relatively inactive has a one in three chance of getting cancer. However, if they are an athlete (or at least active on a regular basis) statistically they'll be in the category of only one case of cancer in seven vastly improving the chance of not getting cancer.

This is largely down to building a strong immune system through the quality of diet and regular exercise. Poor quality of diet is associated with increased risks of many types of cancer*3.

This is one reason it is essential that we start 'tricking' kids into becoming more active and consuming a better diet leading them into losing weight naturally. Overweight children don't like conventional exercise for several reasons. Often they are too large to be good at a sport this means if they are forced into it we are setting them up for failure and making them unhappy.

'...LOSING WEIGHT IS PAINLESS WHEN YOU'RE HAVING FUN.'

Athletes don't choose a sport because they necessarily enjoy it in itself, they choose a sport that makes them feel good because they are good at it. Athletes don't carry on with a sport they are poor at!

This is the same with overweight children. Find an activity they enjoy and it won't seem like a chore or a grueling way to lose weight. We are all aware of how 'time flies when you are having fun' a similar dictum could be said of losing weight. 'Losing weight is painless when you're having fun'.

Another reason that overweight kids avoid exercise and are often bad at conventional sports is because their weight causes some level of low self esteem. It is unlikely that anyone can be good at a sport if they feel self conscious, or have little self worth. We see the effects of this on Champion Athletes all the time. When a sporting failure, or even life situation causes anxiety in an athlete their performance drops and they stop both winning their event and enjoying it.

You are probably fully aware that if you try to force a child into exercising you'll get resistance. This is one reason why I wrote this book. 'Tricking' your child into activity by supplying them with the tools to exercise and lose weight in a fun way is a much more eloquent and painless way to help a kid become healthy.

If you are a parent it is your duty to build your Childs self-esteem and to ensure they have the best quality of life that you can offer them. Being overweight will not help them in any area of their future and it will cause them serious diseases and ultimately a shorter life. On this point I'd also like to mention that studies have shown that if the parents of a Fat child are also over weight themselves it becomes almost impossible for your child to lose weight. So if you are overweight yourself you are going to have to lead by example and start increasing your activity and lose weight. That's the reality of the situation.

'…PREVENTING THEM FROM DYING YOUNG FROM HEART DISEASE OR DIABETES.'

I have outlined in this book fun activities that burn large amounts of Calories and build muscle. Activities that parents can get involved in to support their child and make the activity more enjoyable. Yes, you can also have fun doing these activities with your kid and reap the benefits yourself. Not only will this allow *you* to '*trick*' yourself into exercise, but you will also be getting quality time building a better bond with your child as well.

With the escalating trend of Child Obesity, we need to find a solution to get Children to eat more healthily and increase their level of activity. We all know how difficult it is to change a Childs diet. You can't always stop them eating food that is fattening, or bad for them. You may not have too much say in the food they eat at school, or the exercise they partake in during the day and it's often difficult to regulate the sweets they eat when you are not around.

'…A CHILD BORN AFTER THE YEAR 2000 WILL HAVE 50% CHANCE OF GETTING CANCER IN ADULTHOOD.'

Several generations ago we didn't have this problem. Children played outside, running around burning calories and maintaining a healthy physique. Today activities favoured by children include sedentary games such as X-boxes, TV, the Internet and increasingly Mobile Phone applications.

The solution then is to find fun activities that burn calories and build muscle so their hearts remain strong and they lose weight. Essentially preventing them from dying young from heart disease, cancer or diabetes.

Unfortunately tying them to the wardrobe and force feeding them is frowned upon these days and Intravenous drips are just far too time consuming. So this book aims to give you (humane) ways to trick the little buggers!

It's not just about losing weight, but stopping a child from gaining even more!

If your child does not want to lose weight, or more to the point, resists cutting out their favourite high calorie snack then '*Tricking*' them into enjoying exercising without realising it and replacing their poor diets (particularly snacks) with healthier choices is the best option.

Chapter One - The Reality of Obesity in Kids

The number of overweight school children in the World is around Two Hundred Million [1] (200,000,000) of which Fifty Million are classed as Obese.

Out of these statistics two million overweight school aged children are from the United Kingdom, with a gender ratio of 25% of girls and 20% of boys [2] being overweight.

The United States doesn't fare any better.

In the USA around Twenty Five *Million* kids are overweight with twelve and a half million of those children considered obese *3. That's over thirty percent of the adolescent population. Childhood obesity is unlikely to get any better if a childs parents are overweight *4. Currently seventy two percent of adult men and sixty four percent of adult women are overweight, with about one-third of adults being obese *5.

As a result of this trend, diseases related to being overweight are prominent and often carried over into adulthood. This is the first generation of children in history of whom a large percentage are expected to die before their parents from weight issues.

Some of the issues affecting fat kids are outlined below.

Diabetes in Kids

Diabetes Mellitus is a group of metabolic diseases in which a person has high blood sugar levels either because the body does not produce insulin, or because the body resists the insulin that it does produce.

The main two forms of diabetes that we are interested in are Type 1 (*insulin-dependent diabetes*) and Type 2 (*insulin resistant diabetes*)

In the past Type 1 Diabetes was termed '*Childrens Diabetes'* as it was most often seen in children who had inherited the likelihood of becoming Diabetic. This form of Diabetes is considered to be caused primarily by genetic predispositions.

In contrast, Type 2 diabetes was often labeled '*Adult Diabetes'* because adults were prone to it through diet and lifestyle issues. It was thought children simply hadn't had sufficient time leading a poor lifestyle to develop this type of Diabetes. This has now changed. Kids are now developing Type 2 Diabetes due to poor diets and inactivity and it now accounts for around Ninety Percent of Diabetic cases *6.

A change in diet and activity levels will assist in preventing a child from developing Type 2 Diabetes.

There are also currently Seventy Eight Million (78,000,000) adult Americans suffering from Pre-Diabetes (a staggering 35 percent of the population). Unless some serious changes are made in both adult and children's lifestyles, Diabetes is going to continue to grow.

Heart Disease in Children

Heart disease is the largest cause of death in the United States and the United Kingdom. It is still rarely seen in children however, the risks are increasing due to the growing rate of obese children.

Coronary heart disease is caused when a child consumes too much fat in their diet. Fat builds up in the coronary arteries and the hearts blood supply is blocked. This is when a heart attack may occur.

Changes in a childs diet and activity level can prevent heart disease and strengthen the heart muscle.

Hypertension in Children

Hypertension, or as it is more commonly known 'high blood pressure' is increased blood pressure that can occur in two forms.

There is always an increase in pressure when the heart forces blood into the vessels in order to circulate the body and a lowering of pressure between heart pumps. There is also a constant level of pressure caused from the pressure of the blood against the arteries as the blood flows.

Hypertension is an elevated amount of pressure that the blood is exerting upon the blood vessel walls as the heart pumps above what is usually termed normal.

In children this is also directly related to being overweight from a poor life style and again can be rectified by changing their diet and level of physical activity.

One study [7] by Brenner Children's Hospital found that even with the addition of medication, obese children still retained higher blood pressure than those whose weight was in the healthy range. Therefore, medication is not a valid solution but weight loss is.

Thyroid Damage in Kids

The Thyroid is important in children because it releases the hormones that regulate metabolism and growth. An Italian study [8] found that fat excess in children damages and inflames thyroid tissue. It was previously thought that overweight people had Thyroid problems that caused their weight problems. However, it is now understood that the opposite is true; being overweight as a child causes the Thyroid problems and malfunction.

Sleep Apnoea in Overweight Kids

Sleep Apnoea are brief pauses in breathing during sleep. Often associated with people over fifty years of age and usually due to some form of obstruction in the air waves causing a decrease in oxygen levels such as the build up of fatty deposits. The main symptom being sleepiness during the day as the patient has not had the required 'deep' sleep necessary to rest fully.

Occasionally a normal weight child will suffer sleep Apnoea due to large tonsils and adenoids. This is usually rectified through surgical removal of the Tonsils.

In recent years there has been an increase in the occurrence of childhood Sleep Apnoea thought to be due to the increase in child obesity and Type 2 lifestyle Diabetes*9 and the problem escalates.

Unlike Sleep Apnoea in adults, sleepiness is not observed in children with Apnoea. Instead they display ADD type behaviour which is often incorrectly diagnosed.

Twenty Five percent of overweight children may have sleep problems that regular physical activity can resolve *10. The knock on effect of this is seen in every area of a childs life – social, educational and personal. Not getting the required 'deep' sleep is extremely problematic for a child.

Social Aspects of Child Obesity

There are many social and psychological issues associated with children being overweight. Depression, low self esteem, poor academia and lack of social interaction, as well as having to deal with bullying! These can and will carry on over to adulthood. Poor academia often results in problematic employment opportunities which could lead to life-long problems.

Scarce childhood social interaction may result in a lack of social skills as an adult hindering every area of the kids adult life.

'…A CHILD BORN AFTER THE YEAR 2000 WILL HAVE 50% CHANCE OF GETTING CANCER IN ADULTHOOD.'

Cancer

Due to the obesity problem among children today, it is predicted that a child born in the year 2000 will have a one in two chance of suffering from cancer when an adult *11. Poor diet is directly associated with many forms of cancer.

Chapter Two - Weight Loss for Kids

The foundation of an active lifestyle and a happy life in general is down to the way we fuel our bodies. By consuming a good diet we not only become more energetic but feel stronger in body and mind, become less depressed and are able to cope with the psychological stresses of everyday life. In Children the quality of food is even more important because as they grow the food they eat is setting up their bodies to be healthy and strong during adulthood or weak and ill.

Most people are aware that the easiest route to losing weight is to both burn more calories and to consume fewer calories, from better quality foods in smaller quantities. However, because children may still be growing their dietary requirements are in some ways more important than that of an adult.

Children under five require enough calories and nutrients to allow them to grow, but in small amounts on a regular basis to give their stomachs the time to process the food.

Age and the type of diet is important. Under five year olds require five to ten percent less Protein in the diet than that of over five year olds and around five to fifteen percent more Fat.*1

Large amounts of fibre-rich food is also a bad idea for young children because it can act to fill them up early in a meal (or before a meal), preventing them from consuming more important nutritious foods that their bodies require to grow.

This book is not written with children below five years old in mind, although some scientists *2 are claiming obesity often initiates at two years old and shockingly many babies are now actually being born slightly overweight.

Most of the activities to 'trick' your child into losing weight are not appropriate for the under fives.

Body Fat and Calories in Children

A part of the problem with weight loss in children who are already overweight is that even if they cut the amount of calories they consume they still have vast stores of fat that need burning. This is one of the reasons an overweight child should increase their daily activity. Not only does this burn fat fast, the building of muscle continues to burn calories for around 48 hours after the activity, even at night whilst they are asleep.

For adults it is quite simple to work out the required daily calorific intake and expenditure.

A daily calorie intake for men is about two and a half thousand and two thousand calories per day for women *3.

Children on the other hand, require different levels of calories depending on their age, size, developmental stage and activity level.

On average, under five year olds require around one thousand to two thousand calories per day compared to over five year old children requiring one thousand four hundred to three thousand two hundred calories per day *4.

'...MUSCLE CONTINUES TO BURN CALORIES 48 HOURS AFTER THE ACTIVITY.'

If your child is not involved in much activity it is easy to tell how many calories he or she is over indulging in by monitoring the weight they gain or lose each week. Three and a half thousand calories equals about One pound of fat. So if they are gaining one pound of weight on a weekly basis they are consuming around five hundred calories per day too much! To stop this they must either cut down by at least five hundred calories per day, change the quality of food they consume or increase their activity to burn the excess calories.

The quality of food is important and it is a great way to '*trick*' your child into losing weight without them realising it!

'... IT IS A GREAT WAY TO '*TRICK*' YOUR CHILD INTO LOSING WEIGHT WITHOUT REALISING IT!'

The reason the quality of food is important to weight loss or calorie counting is because different foods supply different amounts of calories (units of energy).

Protein and Carbohydrates provide four calories per gram.

Fats are the 'bad guys' providing the most amount of calories per gram of food at nine calories per gram. Consequently the easiest way to cut down on calories is to substitute fats for protein or carbohydrates in a kids diet.

Consuming Proteins and Carbohydrates rather than Fats has another knock-on effect. If a Kid eats too many calories in this instance the body needs to convert the Protein or Carbohydrates into fat stores, this process in itself requires the burning of additional calories, hence less fat is stored. Where-as Fat is converted instantly with little processing required.

How to Tell if a Kid is Overweight

We saw in the Introduction that many parents do not recognize that their kid is overweight or even Obese! For this reason their needs to be a globally recognized measurement of weight and health. Body Mass Index (BMI) is such a measurement. BMI can be used to measure children or adults however, unlike BMI for adults, BMI for kids is age and gender specific due to their varying growth rates. It is not only used to measure overweight Children but normal and underweight kids too. Measurements are calculated using height and weight. Charts are used to establish whether a kid is over, underweight or at the correct weight.

There are hundreds of kid BMI calculators online which makes the calculations simple. Simply type in 'body mass index calculator for kids' to a search engine, add a kids height, weight and age and you will be presented with the results.

A Balanced Diet for Kids.

Children need a good selection from a variety of foods throughout the day. This will not only give a child the energy and nutrients to grow and maintain health but allow them to think clearly by feeding the brain. Breakfast is the most important meal of the day and we will see later how you can feed them almost anything during breakfast because you cannot get fat from the first meal of the day *5.

Overweight and obese children can almost always benefit from reducing the fat in their diet, or more importantly substitute it for better quality food sources. Parents should consult a doctor or dietician to get specific advice for individual circumstances.

Fats are not all bad, fats from milk for instance has proven to have little effect upon obesity and the benefits are too great to eliminate from a kids diet. Calcium and Vitamin D for instance are difficult to consume in other ways so a daily intake of low fat milk is advised for young children *6.

If your child is going to consume fat it should be from foods that all contain other nutrients like oily fish and red meat rather than empty calories from junk food such as cakes and candy.

The best diet for us all is a balanced diet. Not only will it supply us with the correct nutrition, but keep us lean and stop us becoming too bored with the same old food.

This is not a book about nutrition, but it is essential to gain a little insight into the food groups in order to be able to 'trick' your child into eating a better diet. Primarily by substituting some of their bad food sources with more healthy foods without them realising their diet has become healthy!

The Five Main Food groups

1 - Bread and Starchy foods,

These provide energy, fibre, vitamins and minerals.
Such as cereals, potatoes, rice, pasta, bread.
Choose wholegrain varieties whenever you can.

At least 4 servings per day.

2 - Fruit and vegetables.

Providing fibre, vitamins and minerals and important antioxidants.

1-2 different fruits per day and 5 different vegetables over the day, preferably of different colours (mixing colours is an easy way to know you are supplying a variety of nutrients).

3 - Milk and dairy foods.

A good source of calcium for bone growth and healthy teeth. A good source of protein for muscle and connective tissue growth in children, plus vitamins and minerals.

Dairy products include the following foods; milk, cheese, yoghurt, custard and ice cream (or calcium fortified soy alternatives). At least three servings per day.

4 - Meat, fish, eggs and beans.

A variety of foods stuff which provide mainly protein, but also vitamins and minerals (particularly iron).
Includes meats (beef, lamb, pork and chicken), fish, eggs, pulses, nuts and legumes. For children, try to spread these out through the day, perhaps one serving at lunch and another at dinner.

5 - Foods that contain fat and sugar.

Any food that is fatty, sugary and usually processed is probably bad for a child. These include biscuits, cakes, fizzy drinks, chocolate, sweets, crisps and pastries. We will look at alternatives to these later. Cutting out all fat from your childs diet is not always a good idea. If they are overweight and continue to consume more calories than they burn their body will still store these calories as fat.

Choosing fats from oil and spreads can become slightly complicated because there are good and bad fats. A nice way of remembering as a rough guide is the fats that are bad for you are usually solid at room temperature and contain little nutrition or fiber. These are saturated and/or *Trans* fatty acids. Such as beef fat (suet), butter, cream, chicken fat, pork fat (lard) and margarine.

Polyunsaturated and monounsaturated vegetable oils & spreads are the best types of oil to cook with (such as olive, sunflower and peanut oil).

Kids and Meal Times

Meal times, particularly the evening meal, are the foundation of family life. It is a time when the adults have the opportunity to find out what their kids have been doing during the day, their worries and anxieties and generally support them in life. It's a great opportunity to get together around a table so that all members can talk and listen without other distractions.

There are two other benefits to the overweight child in eating around a table with the family;

One; talking distracts overweight children from focusing on the food that they eat. If they are distracted they are far less likely to be fussy about their food, and are less focused on taste sensation. So it's beneficial to try to make meals times more about the family than the food that you eat.

Two; talking around a meal table prevents diners from eating too quickly. We know that overweight people generally eat much faster than healthy individuals and this prevents the diner's brain from sending the message that it is full and to stop eating! Consequently, fast eaters eat beyond the amount they require before their brains are able to stop them.

Overweight kids often eat far too quickly. Research shows that our bodies take twenty minutes to signal that we are full. The satiety signal is the sensation of being full; it is instigated by the brains Hypothalamus. Humans can feel full and feel hungry simultaneously. Hunger is the physiological need to eat including hunger pangs which are created by the Liver.

'HUMANS CAN FEEL FULL AND HUNGRY SIMULTANEOUSLY.'

The reason it takes twenty minutes for the brain to tell us to stop eating is because it is not the stomach that sends the message to the brain. It is the intestines. Consequently the stomach is already full by the time the intestines have received enough food from the stomach to instigate the message *7.

Eating slower really does mean eating less and still feeling full.

Breakfast

We know that missing breakfast is associated with kids being overweight *8. We know that breakfast 'kick-starts' the body's metabolism following a nutrition 'fast' during a nights sleep, encouraging the body to burn calories immediately after breakfast. If breakfast is missed the body will not burn many calories until the next meal. Therefore, breakfast is vital for weight loss. Missing breakfast also encourages a child to snack mid morning and often on junk food.

Tip; Missing Breakfast reduces your childs ability to concentrate later in the morning and encourages them to feel bad tempered *9.

Breakfast in itself is an aid to weight loss. In fact your child is better off eating a high calorie breakfast than any other meal because it will give your child enough energy to be more active during the day and burn it off *10.

If a Kid is not hungry at breakfast they probably ate too many calories, too late, the night before.

Tip; give your child a glass of milk or fruit juice ten minutes before breakfast, this will help fill them up and give them extra important nutrients and energy for the day ahead. Additionally if your child is eating cereal for breakfast, fruit juice enhances the body's ability to absorb the Iron in the cereal *11.

The best types of breakfast for an overweight child;

Cereals

As a general rule there are two types of cereal, High (nutrient) density cereal and low density. In other words the amount of nutrition packed into the same weight of cereal. Nutrient dense food are usually also low in calories, hence will help a child lose weight, but retain the nutrition that they need to grow. There are of course, foods that are in between high and low density, foods that contain good quality vitamins and minerals but also an average amount of calories.

Don't get too hung up on calories for the breakfast meal, you can't get fat from this meal *12.

Eating some nutrient dense foods, although low in calories may encourage your child to eat more calories per meal. Here is why. Dried Fruit for instance, is high nutrient dense, but will contain more calories per gram than the same fresh fruit because the (non calorific) water has been removed from dried fruit. As a result you are likely to eat more dried fruit than fresh fruit (which means more calories per meal). The nutrients are condensed, your child eats more to satisfy their hunger. However, the food doesn't contain much fat which is really the 'bad guy' in a Childs diet.

Oat Porridge

Porridge oats are a sustained release which means they release their nutrients slowly throughout the day causing your child to remain fuller longer. Whole grain cereals such oatmeal have plenty of complex carbohydrate which maintains consistent energy throughout the day. Porridge also helps lower Cholesterol.

Tip: Add local Honey instead of sugar to sweeten. Local Honey (rather than from another area) has the added effect of making your child more resilient to local pollen if they are prone to allergies and hay fever.) Seek medical advice if you are unsure of a childs allergies.

Rolled Oat Porridge can be a bit of a chore. Some people prefer to prepare it the night before and reheat so that it is quicker in the morning. However, there are some excellent Quick 'microwave' style Porridge style oats designed for Kids that take just two minutes to cook. They are low in fat and have virtually no salt.

Tip; If you have a slow cooker, breakfast oats can be left to cook overnight taking the pain out of preparing oats.

Pitta Breads

Wholemeal is best. High in carbohydrates, low in fat. Watch out for salt as they have a high content of sodium. Pitta breads are quick to prepare in a toaster and due to the pocket style design fun for kids to fill themselves. Encouraging the kids to fill with a selection of healthy fillings will again distract them from whether this is the type of food they want to eat and focus their attention on the enjoyment of preparing and consuming.

A few healthy filling ideas for Pitta breads;

- A great way to slip in some healthy vegetables 'under the radar'!
- Easy to add high protein low fat meats such as Turkey slices or Chicken.

- Cheese (melted or otherwise), lettuce, tomato and cucumber etc
- Add Hummus, roasted peppers, cucumbers, mushrooms etc

Tip: Turkey is not only high in protein and low in fat it is also the only meat that helps elevate the mood. It has 'feel' good qualities because it contains an amino acid called Tryptophan. Tryptophan is converted into 5 hydroxytryptophan (5-HTP) which is then converted to Serotonin – the feel good hormone!

Scrambled Eggs

The key to healthy scrambled eggs is to not to add too much butter and keep to low fat milk. In fact, although butter makes it more creamy most kids won't notice if you leave it out. Ultimately it depends on the child, if they need the energy requirements from butter in the morning there is no harm in adding it.

Poached eggs are also a quick way to cook eggs and healthier than scrambled eggs as no additional ingredient is required. They can be easily placed on a piece of rustic brown bread for a quick breakfast. *More egg ideas are in the next section.*

Homemade Smoothies

Quick and easy. Use semi-skimmed or coconut milk. Having prepared ingredients is the key and a good selection dependant on your childs taste.

Try pre-frozen banana, melon and berries for plenty of fruit to start the day. Add Yogurt if desired.

Try not to add sugar, again honey or syrup is usually better to sweeten.

There are thousands of smoothie and shake recipes on the Internet that you can download.

Tip: If Mum and Dad want to join in but 'need' their morning caffeine blast! Try a Coffee Smoothie with real instant coffee, banana and ice blended together.

Lunch

Controlling what kids consume at lunch can be difficult when they are attending school. Of course, even if you have taught them what constitutes healthy food it doesn't mean that they are going to go down that route! Packed lunches are an easier way to control what they consume during the day.

Don't let them get too bored with mundane sandwiches. There are so many different types of breads, wraps, bagels, Rye bread and Pittas many of which are available as whole grain. They could have something different each day of the week! Again use the Internet for ideas, simply typing in 'healthy sandwich ideas for kids' brings up pages of school lunch ideas.

Turkey-Meatball Pitas

Lean Meatballs are a great healthy alternative to the familiar more fattening beef meatballs which many children find comforting. Using Turkey as a healthy alternative meat means your child is likely not to feel a sense of loss from the fattening food they once ate.

Advantages of healthy Meat Balls;

- Extra convenient enveloped in a Pitta.

- Goes well with almost any vegetable for extra nutrition.

- Onions, peppers, lettuce, tomatoes are easy to add.

- You can even mix up your own sauce to go with it.

Tuna

If like many Kids yours don't like, or eat much fish, Tuna is often a good solution that may also slip 'under the radar' as being healthy. Tinned Tuna doesn't have bones and is easily mixed with low calorie mayonnaise, sweet corn and many other additives. Tuna is very versatile and a great source of protein and omega oils. It can be added to a small pot of salad, into sandwiches, with Pasta to form a pasta bake with crushed crisps on top to add something more familiar to a Kids experience.

Eggs

Eggs are a very healthy versatile food. Hard boiled eggs are easy to transport and keep in the fridge for some time. Depending on the age of your child, you can cut boiled eggs in to funny shapes or faces as a part of a main meal.

When boiling an egg you can add food colouring to surprise your child with a pink or red egg inside!

If your kids don't like eggs, dressing them up in bread crumbs could be a way to enhance the flavour.

A scrambled egg can be wrapped in a flour tortilla with the addition of some secretly placed lettuce or vegetables to 'trick' your kid into gaining some bonus nutritional value! Easily added to a lunch box.

Pasta

Small pots of pasta can be added to a packed lunch. Add Olives, vegetables, Avocado or anything that your child enjoys. Mix small chunks of meat to add protein, ham or turkey perhaps.

Low calorie sauces are a plenty. Just search the internet to make your own.

Dinner / Evening Meal

As stated earlier in this Chapter, Dinner is best served with the whole family preferably seated around a table. This setting offers many benefits;

- Enhanced family communication.
- Distraction from food for fussy eaters.

- The reduction of eating pace (so fewer calories are consumed during one sitting).
- Enables parents to discretely monitor a childs food consumption and eating habits.
- Enables parents and siblings to support an overweight child in eating healthily.

Disguising Food

Using a vegetable that perhaps your Kid doesn't like and disguising it with a food they do like is a great way of 'tricking' them into losing weight. A lot of Kids don't like Broccoli sprouts for instance but they do like Cauliflower Cheese. Green vegetables like Broccoli are extremely important to growing kids. They are high in antioxidants and Broccoli is good for the digestive tract assisting with detoxing the body. So adding Broccoli in with the Cauliflower and cooking with cheese might be a way of getting your kid eating quality green food. The cheese maybe slightly high in fat but you have to weigh up the Pro's and Con's of all the foods.

Weight Loss and the Household Environment

To support a Kid in weight loss you need to set the environment up for Success! They can't eat it, if you don't have it in the House! Of course don't just throw all the 'bad' food away in the house, that would be wasteful. Just stop replenishing it, let it run out organically.

Keep convenient healthy alternatives at hand. You might be surprised at how many carrot sticks your kid will eat if they're readily available with a tasty Dip as an accompaniment! Dips can be easily and inexpensively made with healthy ingredients. Fruit slices to dip into Yogurt. A dish of Peanut butter with slices of toast to dip. You can use almost any fruit or vegetable sliced into sticks or chunks. *See the next section for some ideas.*

Remember kids copy their parents, if you are leaving chocolate bar wrappers around the house whilst advising the kids to eat a piece of fruit it isn't going to work. Lead by example!

Consider both the household environment and the behaviour of your kids. If they rush home from school and go immediately to turn the TV on, leave a healthy snack by the chair that they sit on whilst watching TV.

Watch your kids undesirable behaviour, when they attack the fridge for a snack for instance, try to interrupt that behaviour.

Tip; Interrupting behaviour patterns is a well known technique used by Psychologists to create change in people. If you can interrupt this pattern of behaviour and replace it with a more desirable one your child will change.

Protein Snacks for Kids

Eggs

We've already mentioned eggs. But it's worth noting that as a snack they can be excellent. Pickled eggs keep "forever" and there is no reason why you shouldn't slice them into small segments, add some onion and a cocktail stick and serve as a snack. Eggs are popular used as Hors d'oeuvres. For instance, Scrambled Eggs wrapped in Salmon, an extremely high protein snack with the benefits of an oily fish! It is a great way to 'trick' a kid into substituting crisps and candy for high quality food.

Honey

Add to cereal, fruit, drinks as an alternative to sugar. Get some local honey in for the cupboard!

Hummus

Hummus is a popular high protein Middle Eastern

dip, easy to make yourself out of chickpeas or garbanzo beans. Plenty of recipes on the Internet.

As with all dips you can 'dunk' almost anything. Chunks of cheese, toast slices or gets those greens in again with broccoli florets, cauliflower and carrot sticks.

Milkshakes

Milkshakes are similar to smoothies. The main difference is a milkshake is a blend of milk and or ice cream, with added flavours usually in the form of syrup. A smoothie is a mixture of fruit, ice and either fruit juice, water and yogurt. Of course Milkshakes are less nutritious than smoothies however *you* are in charge, you can add whatever you wish. If a child requires extra protein and calcium in their diet low fat milk in a Milkshake is an easy way to feed it to them.

Nuts and Seeds

Nuts and seeds are high protein foods. Easily transported and come in a huge selection of types. Experiment and see which type your kid prefers. Some nuts are high in fat. However, it is Monounsaturated fat which helps to raise your "good" cholesterol while at the same time lowering your "bad" cholesterol.

Salted peanuts are of course not ideal due to the added salt however if that's the only way your Child will eat nuts then the pro's may outweigh the con's? It's up to you to get individual advice on this. An alternative to salted nuts are dry roasted and raw unroasted nuts. Roasting nuts loses some of the nutritional value and some of the calorific content from the monounsaturated fats. Roasted nuts are considered by many to taste better, which is probably something most Kids agree with. So you or your child needs to weigh up if taste or nutrition is most important.

Nuts are an easy snack to leave in a bowl. Of course there are some kids with Nut allergies, obviously avoid in this case. In addition small children can choke on nuts so make sure your kids are old enough and supervised.

Seeds are also great sources of protein, minerals, zinc and other nutrients. Numerous studies have shown that different types of seeds can actually prevent weight gain, the development of heart disease and the accumulation of LDL (bad) cholesterol.

They also come in a huge variety of types and tastes. Again roasted or not, organic or not etc.

Tofu

Tofu is packed with protein. In most cases you will need to 'trick' your child into eating it. Add strong flavours. Low fat Tofu kebabs with peppers and Chicken or Turkey is a great way of disguising this healthy food.

Noodles with tofu and vegetables in a spicy sauce is also a great 'trick' to encourage a kid into consuming nutritious ingredients.

High Energy Foods and Drinks for Kids

When dieting, the reduction in the vast amount of sugary foods that a child has become accustomed to may result in a need for additional energy boosting snacks. Especially if an increase in calorie burning activity is planned (which it is!).

Energy boosters can be in the form of foods or drinks.

Baked Beans.
Baked Beans and Cheese on Toast is an old favorite, full of Carbohydrates, Protein in the Beans and Cheese. Grate the cheese for flavour so that you use it sparingly. Depending on the cheese it maybe high in fat.
Baked Potato and Baked Beans are easy to prepare by precooking. If you oven cook the potato, you can simple reheat it later with the beans. If you have a Microwave then it's only a ten minute job anyway.

Bananas
Firm favourite of Athletes. Quick burst of energy

after consumption, easy to transport, they even come in their own portable case! Full of antioxidants, vitamin C, high in simple and complex carbohydrates and fibre.

Plain yoghurt

Easily transported and stacked with Protein and Carbohydrates for energy. Add crushed cereal on top for an extra boost of energy and flavour.

Popcorn

Probably not a food you'll have to trick your child into eating, so don't tell them that Popcorn is a healthy wholegrain! High in Dietary fibre in the form of energy-producing complex carbohydrates , low in fat and calories.

Popcorn has a bad reputation due to the high calorie buttered or salted varieties you find at your local cinema. Stay clear of this type. Get the unsalted and unbuttered, or better still invest in a popcorn making machine and get the kids involved! A great, healthy way to distract them from eating junk before their main meal.

Powdered Milk

Mixing a few spoons of powdered milk to milk drinks can enhance the energy effects, protein and nutrients. Use lower fat milks to keep the calories down.

Adding powdered milk to cooking can also increase the energy and protein content without your child being aware of it.

Drinks

Cola (and other canned drinks) are usually full of sugar and contain caffeine, neither of which are desirable for an overweight child.

Try making your own fizzy drinks. Drinks makers are quite inexpensive these days and last for years. This is a great way of knowing what each bottle of drink you give a child contains without checking every label. You can add whatever it is that you want your child to consume.

This is probably one of the best ways to get your child to drink water without the diuretic effects of caffeine.

Drinks with natural sugar such as fruit juices are another quick way of boosting the energy for your child. Be careful not to buy the ones with additives. Again purchasing a fruit squeezer is the best way to know what's in your childs drink and you can enroll your kid into doing the squeezing, simultaneously educating them in foods and tastes.

Buying fizzy drinks makers and orange squeezers are a long term investment and will save you money in the long run. Not to mention the benefits to the long term health of your child in which you do need to *INVEST*.

Chapter Three - How to Trick a Kid into Weight Loss

The whole concept of this book is about tricking Kids into having fun without realising that they are exercising, burning Calories and reducing their body fat. This Chapter offers more detailed strategies to do this seamlessly.

Don't Pressurise Your Kids

Pressurising a child or an adult for that matter, only leads to resistance. Creating resentment in your child won't do much for your relationship and definitely won't help them lose weight.

Lead by example and they will pick up your behaviours, habits and attitude. Without being aware of it you'll be tricking them into learning about healthy food and nutrition.

If they ask questions like "why have we no crisps?" in the house or "why have we so much fruit in the Kitchen", state that you are feeling much happier since eating extra fruit, that it's healthy and you have much more energy and vitality eating those sorts of foods.

Focus your answers onto whatever it is that is important to your child. If being more active is something they aspire to then mention those traits in yourself. If they wish to do better at school, mention that since eating more vegetables your mind is clearer, your memory is better or you can concentrate at work better than before perhaps.

You know your child best so focus on the traits you think will LEVERAGE change in them.

Distraction and Taste Sensation

We've already touched upon this in previous chapters and it's a technique most Mothers of babies are familiar with. When a baby cries, the first thing most mothers do is distract them from the source of the problem.

It's the same with overweight kids. We are not talking about using a TV as distraction – your child will just eat faster and pay less attention to their full signals.

Tip; An athlete doesn't focus on taste but gains as much pleasure from food as an overweight person. An Athlete focuses on the Freshness and Crunchiness of a Carrot, for instance and how it benefits their body.

We're talking about stimulating their minds with conversation during a meal so that the food becomes less of a focus or an issue. We're talking about disguising some foods that are healthy if they'd otherwise not eat them. We're talking about directing their attention to the benefits of healthier foods in relation to what is important in their own lives.

We want them to focus less on taste sensation and more on the benefits of good quality food. Many overweight people *fear* the loss of certain comfort foods, the fear that they will lose the pleasure they get from food if they change to a healthy diet. An athlete doesn't focus on taste but gains as much pleasure from food as an overweight person. An Athlete focuses on the Freshness and Crunchiness of a Carrot, for instance.

The way the freshness is fuelling his or her body for performance. They FEEL the energy in their body, they FEEL great about themselves that they are building their bodies and their future. As they eat they imagine their bodies getting stronger – it excites them to 'feel' the changes!

Other ways to distract your Kids;

Food of the Week.
Try a new food every week? We know from kids with eating disorders, food often becomes an important issue in their lives along with negative emotions and

anxiety. The more relaxed you can approach food the more relaxed a child should be. Having fun with food can both educate and transform a 'painful' issue or obsession in to a relaxed enjoyable experience. Experiencing a new food or snack once a week can help to add additional nutrients to a childs diet without them realising it. It can help get them involved in the selection of food every week including allowing them to research the internet or local ethnic shops that they'd previously been unfamiliar.

This doesn't have to be a whole different meal but perhaps a different type of nut, fruit, vegetable, spice, condiment or just a new cooking ingredient.

Themed Meals.

Similar to the above 'Food of the week', but a whole experience! Food from other cultures is a good way to add unusual nutrients to your kids diet. Learning about different cultures food, ingredients, ways of cooking and even lifestyles. Get them to dress-up in authentic national dress of said culture perhaps. It is an excellent way to distract your child from the loss of their usual fattening diet and 'trick' them into eating healthily.

Starter (1st Course)

Offering a 'starter', or two course meal may seem a little 'high brow' but there is method in the madness.

We've already mentioned that it takes around twenty minutes for a kids brain to signal that they are full and need to stop eating. For this reason a starter five minutes before the main meal will get your childs stomach breaking down the food and instigating the 'I am full' mechanism way before the main meals is consumed. In addition if you select a 'starter' that is slow to eat such as a light soup, all the better!

Plate Design

Smaller Plates - Purchasing smaller plates will 'trick' your child into selecting less food and still feel they have eaten plenty (as they had a full plate).

Red Plates and Cups – Research [1] claiming red plates instigate an ancient fear response in humans and make them eat less. The theory is that as more of the red colour is exposed on the plate (when food is eaten) the increasingly exposed red colour unconsciously saturates the mind making the diner feel less of an inclination to carry on eating. The report in the Journal Appetite reported over forty percent reduction in consumption of food and drink.

Educating your Kids to Cook.

Studies have shown that kids who are allowed to be actively involved in preparing meals and snacks become more interested in healthier food and nutrition. This interest can only increase if they are encouraged to 'stamp their mark' on the food that they have helped to prepare.

Depending on their age, allowing kids to have fun with food, arranging food as a smiling face on the plate for example, will also encourage them to get involved.

Of course encouraging kids to be active in cooking doesn't just stop in the kitchen it extends to meal planning, shopping, and the preparation of food.

The American Dietetic Association state that kids who cook have higher self confidence and sets them up for important life skills for the future.

'...EATING MEALS AS A FAMILY COULD PREVENT A KID FROM BECOMING A DRUG ADDICT!'

A surprising benefit of kids cooking comes from 'The National Center on Addiction and Substance Abuse' at Columbia University. In their report, *Family Matters: Substance Abuse and the American*

Family[2], the center recommends 10 steps parents can take to prevent substance abuse. Among them are 'cooking with the kids' and 'eating a family meal around a table'. So eating meals with the family really could prevent a child from becoming a drug addict!

Changing the Language you use.

It always amazes me how many parents tell their kids that a food is bad for them and the next moment they offer it to them and state that it's a treat! This is confusing for a child who is learning what is good or bad for them. A food that is unhealthy should never be called a treat because treats have connotations that they are desirable. We want kids to learn that unhealthy foods are never desirable and certainly not a treat. After all their hearts won't consider it a treat when the fat from the 'treat' blocks their arteries! I am sure you have similar terms that you use which are contradictory, be aware of these.

It is not just the words parents use that send confusing messages. Behaviour does the same thing. Kids model all behaviours and that includes good (or bad) eating habits. Make sure yours are sending the desired message. There is little point telling a child to eat their Greens when you have left yours!

Encourage your Child by making health focused comments about food you'd like them to eat even if it's a food that they currently do not enjoy. Amusing comments make the greatest impact, humour is an excellent way for kids and adults to learn. Perhaps whilst eating carrots you mention how wonderful they are because they help you see in the dark. Or the age old one that Spinach will make you strong like Popeye the sailor! How many children have forced down spinach in the past just to get big and strong like Popeye?!

Substituting the worst offenders.

It doesn't take much thought to 'trick' your child into eating more healthily by substituting some of the worst foods that they eat with healthier versions.

Many Colas are bad for kids in a multitude of ways and they do cause weight gain. You can of course substitute a carbonated drink such as cola for something completely different such as a Smoothie or Milkshake. However, kids are creatures of habit and the addiction to fizzy drinks might be difficult to break. It is much easier to make your own drinks with healthy ingredients. We've already mentioned drinks machines such as Sodastream whose nutritional content is vastly more healthy than most canned drinks. If you're not convinced checkout the Soda Stream website for nutrition comparison charts of all the main canned drinks. You might be surprised at the differences.

Rewind the Corporate Brainwashing

Pepsi Cola didn't pay Michael Jackson millions of dollars to star in their adverts because they liked his dancing! They paid him because people associate emotionally with his hit songs at an unconscious level. When you hear a song by a popular artist, even if it's just out of conscious awareness in a shop for instance, you start to feel good. You might even start singing along to yourself or dancing without realising it! The songs are emotional triggers, feel good triggers which advertising companies deliberately manipulate to make us feel good about their products.

When a kid see's or hears a celebrity with a can of Pepsi for instance, they initially feel good about the celebrity. They also subconsciously associate the celebrity with the can of drink they have and then 'anchor' that same emotion for the celeb to that drink. The advertiser now has them! They will feel good every time they see the can of drink and probably buy it.

Why do you think Nike now uses just a symbol (the tick sign) to represent its brand rather than its full name of Nike? Because it has managed to connect so many celebrities with the sign, it can now slip the sign into our unconscious minds when we least expect it. Using a sign means that people don't even notice that they are being advertised to by Nike. Because Nike haven't mentioned the name – they just put a tick on a billboard or on a team mates shoe and it goes into our minds.

Can you rewind this brain washing? Some of it perhaps. If you want to wean a child of a caffeine loaded sugary cola, establish powerful emotional anchors yourself with healthier substitutes. If you want to use a Soda-stream, make it fun for a child to choose and make their own drink! Encourage them to make the best flavour, to make the healthiest drink and reward them with praise. There is not a much more powerful emotional anchor for a child than their parents approval!

This is just an example, it is not just drink that advertisers condition us into buying, they do it with everything. So be aware and start conditioning your child yourself!

Join in! (More on this is the next chapter)

One study by the University of California-San Diego *3 found that kids attempting to lose weight found it impossible if their parents were also overweight and not dieting with them. There was a direct association with child weight loss and parental weight loss.

Which means if you are overweight you must join your child in their weight loss campaign or they are set for failure.

Getting involved also means joining in with the activities that they do. There is nothing in the Chapter on 'tricking your kid into exercise' that you can't do with them! Not only will this help you lose weight and become healthier but it can be fun, quality time with your kids.

Chapter Four - How to Trick a Kid into Feeling Great!

The Jury is out, one of the quickest and healthiest ways to feel good about yourself is to exercise. Not only does it saturate the brain with oxygen rich blood so a kid can think clearly, it releases feel good endorphins making a child happier and reducing stress.

Benefits of Exercise

It doesn't matter how young or old you are, how much you weigh, or your level of athletic ability, aerobic exercise is good for you. Not only for your physique but mental health too[*1].

Exercise releases endorphins (the feel good hormones), it helps to feed your brain with fresh oxygenated blood. The problem is that many people have had bad experiences with exercise and associate pain to any type of activity that remotely resembles sport!

'...YOU DON'T HAVE TO BE GOOD AT AN EXERCISE TO ENJOY IT!'

This is one reason why I wrote this book. The growing number of people who are overweight and see no way of escaping that situation is largely due to lack of activity because they hate exercise.

You don't have to be slim to enjoy exercise, you don't have to be good at it! And you don't have to go to a gym or even exercise outside of your own home.

I wrote this book so people could change the way they perceived activity so that they could start to enjoy sports without feeling bad.

Kids must get into the habit of daily physical activity, if that means enjoying a fun activity that they don't consider to be exercise but still gain the same benefits then all the better!

Exercise is the 'miracle cure' that we all need and the good news is it can be free!

'...50% REDUCTION IN RISK OF DEPRESSION.'

Some of the benefits that kids are likely to enjoy throughout their lives from regular exercise are as follows;

- A 30% lower risk of becoming depressed [6]
- 50% lower risk of coronary heart disease and stroke [2]
- 50% lower risk of type 2 Diabetes [2]
- 40 % - 50% lower risk of Colon Cancer [3, 5]

- 20% to 30% lower risk of Breast and Prostate Cancer *4
- Enhanced ability to lose weight and keep it off
- Clearer arteries
- Stronger immune system hence reduce Colds and Flu
- Strengthened Heart
- Increased stamina and endurance
- A prolonged healthy life

How much Exercise?

The UK National Health Service recommends various guidelines of activity for different age groups. As previously mentioned this book is not for under five year olds as their dietary and exercise requirements are different from older kids because they are developing at an exceptionally rapid rate. In addition, activity for under five year olds can be remarkably light such as merely standing still (which does have an effect of burning more calories than sitting down in all age groups). The advice for under five year olds is moderate activity for around three hours per day split up throughout the day*7. Perhaps a little more if the child is overweight.

Children between the ages of five and eighteen in good health should be partaking in at least one hour per day of moderate to intense aerobic activity (more on these types of activities later).

On several days of the week muscle and bone strengthening exercises should be incorporated into a childs activity (these are also discussed in more detail in a subsequent Chapter).

If a child is overweight, these exercise guidelines will help them improve their health even if they don't lose weight. However, overweight children rarely partake in this amount of exercise so the likelihood is that they will reduce their body fat significantly if they do.

An overweight child attempting to lose weight could of course increase this amount of activity and it is highly likely that they will when I show you later how to 'trick' your kid into exercising without realising it!

How a Childs body responds to exercise

Aerobic exercise is often associated with static cycles in Gyms and Aerobic Dance classes however, any activity that increases a childs heart beat and the amount of Oxygen in their blood could be classed as Aerobic. Aerobic is in contrast to anaerobic exercise which is short 'spurt' type exercise such as weight lifting, or sprinting that usually builds muscle. Of course some activities are a mixture of the two.

Any activity that requires kids to move their leg and arm muscles for a prolonged period should be enough to burn fat and improve their health. Breathing will become faster and deeper, the heart will beat faster increasing the body's Oxygen levels.

Intense exercise also helps carry away Carbon Dioxide and other 'waste' products in the blood. The child will release Endorphins to enjoy an elated feeling following exercise.

Understanding exercise intensity

Because we are not promoting conventional exercise here, but tricking a child into exercising by enjoying fun activities that offer the same benefits, it is important to know about Exercise Intensity. There is little point a in child becoming more active if it is not intense enough to burn fat and build muscle. The idea is to turn a fun activity into exercise by increasing the intensity whilst retaining the fun factor.

There is of course a multitude of scientific ways to calculate and monitor exercise intensity however; this book is not aimed at Sports Scientists! So we will keep things simple.

Gauges of Intensity; Perceptions, Heart and Breathing rate.

It doesn't matter how fit or unfit a child is intensity can be viewed as a personal perception. If a child feels as if the exercise is intense then it probably is! Slightly uncomfortable is what we're looking for because with each activity session we're seeking Progression.

According to Dr Gunnar Borg[*8] from The University of Chester, Perceived Exertion, can be measured on a scale of six to twenty, with six on the scale being no exertion and twenty being maximum exertion. The Harvard School of Public Health state[*9] that most moderate-intensity activities correspond to an exertion of between 12 and 15 on Borgs scale.

This is a great way to gauge intensity in your kid when involved in activity. And you don't need to ask them about their level of intensity as you'll be able to see physically. Remember we are aiming to trick your kid into exercise, we don't want them to become aware that this is the intended outcome. It is just a fun activity to them. If your kid is enjoying a game of 'swing ball' for example and not really exerting themselves, you can discretely encourage them to speed the game up. Or if you're playing with them you could up-the-pace yourself until you see that they are breathing more deeply.

More detailed examples of different intensity exercises are in the next Chapter.

'...WE ARE AIMING TO TRICK A KID INTO EXERCISE, WE DON'T WANT THEM BECOMING AWARE OF THE INTENDED OUTCOME!

Beware of over-exerting a child. If they are short of breath rather than breathing deeply, or they have pain of some kind they may be pushing beyond their current fitness level. Although we're looking for progression we're looking for it over weeks not days! As stated in the front of this book, medical advice or advice from a professional exercise specialist should be sought before undertaking any form of exercise or change in diet.

Getting involved

Exercise is no different from dieting in that, parental involvement can only enhance the probability of success.

The best way to teach someone something is to lead by example. Don't just try to encourage your child by telling them to do something because you may hit resistance. Join in and get involved yourself! And let's face it, you're not getting any younger yourself!

Try taking them out at the weekend cross country cycling or hiking. Go somewhere interesting to stimulate their minds too. Go and see an ancient monument for example. Hire a couple of Kayaks, if you don't live by the coast most places have some sort of lake, river or even a swimming pool that offers such facilities.

Chapter Five - How to Trick a Kid into Exercise!

The key to getting overweight kids to exercise is to find Fun Activities that burn large amounts of Calories and Build Muscle.

The British National Health Service recommend[*1] one hour per day of exercise with a mixture of intensities throughout the week.

Calories burned in the following section are based on a child of no more than 120 Ibs (8.5 stones), the amount of Calories burned dramatically increase with increased weight.

Activities that a Tricked Kid will Love

Hula Hooping – Calories burnt = 420 per hour!

A child can do this inside when it's raining so no excuses!

Hoops are quite inexpensive to buy and last for years however, it is relatively easy to make a Hula Hoop from simple 3/4" tubing, getting a kid to make their own hoop is a great way to get them involved and divert their attention away from the fact that this is going to be exercise! Tubing and connectors can be purchased from most DIY or Builders stores.

Heavier Hula Hoops spin slower and burn more calories but most kids will want a lighter one to start with. Hoops are also available in different sizes. As a general rule measure a kid from sternum to the floor for the ideal diameter of the tube.

Decorate the hoop to a Childs taste with coloured tape around the tubing and add beads internally for a noise effect.

More detailed information on making and exercising with Hula Hoops can be found in my book – '***How to Hula Hoop to Lose Weight***' available on Amazon.

Some benefits of Hooping;

- Hoops are Easy and Fun to make
- Multiple tricks to learn
- Easy to up the intensity
- Hoop to music helps dictate a mixture of fast and slow tempo
- Hoop between TV adverts for an Interval type training session!
- Collapsible hoops are available for easy of transportation
- Tones core muscles and massages stomach fat away
- Vigorous Hooping burns a high amount of calories
- Improves mood

- Doesn't seem like exercise!

Pogo-ing – Calories burnt = 600 per hour!

Pogo sticks allow a kid to burn more calories than almost any other activity whilst being great fun. Pogo sticks are a great way to '*trick*' a kid into exercise without them knowing. Builds leg and arm muscles and requires input from all core muscles.

Lots of modern designs now available with the addition of hydraulic assistance for a high hop!

Swimming – Calories burnt = 400 to 500 per hour depending on the 'stroke'.

Not a great activity if your child is body conscious due to being overweight. But never-the-less it is a fun activity that a kid probably won't consider as exercise. It is easy to mix up 'messing around' in the Pool with real swimming of lengths of the pool.

For an even more intense swim take your kid to a river or the sea, swimming against a current is more taxing and burns more Calories. Caution must be used in open water swimming, as there are obvious dangers. Kids should be supervised and a Life Guard monitored stretch of water should be sought.

Interestingly just 'treading water' can burn up to 500 Calories per hour if done vigorously.

Skating – Calories burned Skating = 350 per hour. Skating is a good upper and lower body exercise and encourages good balance. Good Aerobic exercise if done vigorously. Builds firm thigh muscles. More beneficial if arms are swung whilst skating.

Swing Ball – Calories burnt = 600 per hour

Swing ball is a bat and ball game for one or two players. The tennis sized ball is tethered to a spring at the top of a pole (5ft in height) with a helical screw (coil) at the top of the pole. The object of the game is for the two players to hit the ball in a way that their opponent misses the ball. The first to reach the end of the coil (top or bottom) wins.

Swing balls are generally bought rather than made and are available as a 'drive into the ground' based pole or weighted bases that you fill with sand or water. This makes them more indoor friendly.
Good upper body strength building and good for co-ordination. Can be played on own or with a friend. Also a good anaerobic workout working the lower body, back and core muscles.

If played with a friend the game inevitably becomes very demanding as the competitive spirit will undoubtedly be released in the kids. As the intensity increase (and calories burnt) the game becomes more like a fun activity than exercise and the time will pass rapidly.

Tether Ball - Calories burnt = 200 per hour.

Tether ball is very similar idea to Swing ball but this pole is much higher and the object of the game is somewhat different. Tetherball poles are often 10ft high with a Volleyball tethered to the top of the pole. As with Swing ball the object of the game is for the two opponents to hit the ball in opposite directions. But in this case hands are used to hit the ball rather than bats.

The goal is to hit the ball out of the opponents reach until the winning side wraps the rope all the way around the pole.

Poles are easy to make however they are not as convenient as Swing balls in that they are fixed rather than portable and they are much higher and a lot more room is required.

Relatively active game good cardiovascular workout. Builds strong arms and back muscles.

Jump on a Bouncy Castle - Calories burnt = 500 per hour.

Another great activity that will 'slip under the radar' of a kid who doesn't like exercise. No child will realise this is helping them to get fit and burn fat! Not very practical as a lot of room is required and the likelihood of owning one is slim. Small versions can be hired for the weekend alternatively many amusement parks have these as attractions.

Excellent way to have fun and burn fat. Good opportunity for your kid to make friends and socialise. One of the few activities where being overweight is an advantage!

Space Hopper – Calories burnt = 200 per hour.

Another retro toy that has passed 'the test of time'.

A bouncy, sit on inflatable rubber ball with rubber handles on top (usually in the form of animal ears).

Excellent cardiovascular workout and anaerobic exercise for the thigh muscles and forearms (to grip on) also develops both balance and coordination.

Difficult activity to use for long periods and not very good for travelling any distance. But good fun.

Twister - Calories burnt = 200 per hour

An easy one to 'trick' a kid into getting involved as a form of play.

Doesn't look like exercise but due to the fact that participants spend a great deal of time in unusual positions held up often by one or two legs it is a great muscle builder and developer of balance. It depends on the positions that a kid is requested to form as to which muscle groups are developed.

Good for socialising with other kids.

Bowling/Skittles – Calories burnt = 200 per hour

You don't have to spend a fortune visiting a bowling alley! Although that can be fun too. You could of course use anything for Pins and the bowling ball such as soft drink bottles half full of water for pins and a Football for a bowling ball.

Skittle sets are inexpensive and available from toy stores.

The key here is to have fun plus make the activity difficult enough to burn calories, that means a weighted ball if possible to build those shoulder and back muscle (hence burn fat).

Skipping / Rope Jumping – Calories burnt = 860 per hour

Skipping is a favourite of Boxers for good reason - it's a great workout for your heart and lungs and the act of jumping also strengthens bones, which can help to prevent osteoporosis.

Great fitness and co-ordination for boys and girls. Some boys may perceive this as being a bit feminine due to its dominance by girls in the play ground. If you remind them that boxers skip on a daily basis this may encourage them to have a go.

Ropes can be expensive, a child could just use an old piece of rope to reduce the cost. There are many styles of skipping rope available to buy from handles with bearings for a smooth turn to speed ropes and ropes that count the repetitions.

Skipping is great for a variety of reasons not limited to the fact that it burns more Calories than almost any other activity. It can be done with several kids one child at each end of a rope.

Boxing skipping is slightly different from the skipping you see in play grounds. The skipper does not jump high lifting their knees up, but lifts the feet with a slightly raised toe to a level just above the heel.

Tricks such as crossing the rope over whilst in flight offer variety.

More information on skipping for fitness is available in my book '***How to Skip Like a Boxer***' available on my website www.SportsHypnosis.co.uk or on Amazon.

Tai Chi or Yoga – Calories burnt = 200 - 250 per hour

Tai Chi is not always the first choice for a kid looking seeking a new activity but a growing trend. Kids like the connotations it has of the Martial Artist. Good for kids who get stressed.

Builds muscle tone and strength. Relaxes the body and mind. Improves posture, balance and co-ordination.

Reduces anxiety.

Cycling – Calories burnt = 300 - 700 per hour (depending on speed and terrain.)

Cycling is one of the most popular sports in the United Kingdom with an estimated three million cyclists every month partaking.

It is a great way to 'get out of the house' and discover new places. Which why it is a favorite of families looking to spend time together and increase their fitness simultaneously.

Moderate in aerobic benefits if taken at a leisurely pace. Cycle 'off road' on rough terrain or at speed in hilly conditions and it becomes a powerful Aerobic fat burner and muscle building exercise.

Builds endurance in legs and builds strong heart and lungs.

An easy way to vary intensity of exercise in a Child.

Push – ups – Calories burnt = 1 Calorie per push-up (not really an hourly Calorie burner)

A kid is unlikely to spend an hour doing press-ups so the hourly Calorie burning statistic is a little pointless.

However, this is a firm muscle builder and as we know from the previous chapters muscle continues to burn calories for at least 48 hours after the muscle building activity. So it is still an efficient fat burning activity.

An excellent addition to the muscle building weekly routine and a great opportunity for Dad to challenge the kids to a weekly press up competition! Draw a chart and compete every Sunday afternoon for example.

Builds strength in Chest, Arms and Shoulders. Increases muscle endurance. Can also assist in Cardiovascular strengthening if completed in rapid succession.

Zumba – Calories burnt = 350- 800 per hour (depending on intensity and equipment used)

Zumba is the current Dance craze however any form of structured dance routine can be of huge benefit to an overweight Kid.

Zumba is a Latin based music routine popular due to the up-beat nature of the music. I challenge any kid to feel depressed whilst working out in this manner.

Great exercise because it incorporates interval training, in other works switching from fast to slow in pace.

Predominately Aerobic in activity but the addition of props or resistance type equipment such as dumbbells enhances the muscle building potential.

Easy to do at home with a DVD but far more effective in a class environment as motivation is higher and generally classes offer a more fun environment so enjoyment is increase (increasing the likelihood of continuing)

Playgrounds and Adventure Areas – Calories burnt = 400- 500 per hour

When I was a child we were always in the woods somewhere building a den, climbing trees and generally building muscle, outside breathing healthy air. Of course these days there seems to more of a concern for child safety. We didn't wear crash hats when cycling somewhere, but our parents always knew where we were, we checked in on a regular basis and they knew who we were with (usually in groups of three or four as a minimum). So we remained relatively safe. Ok we had the odd injury, but boys will be boys! People don't 'grow' if you don't let them make some mistakes in life.

Kids (depending on their age) love to climb things. Whether it's a climbing frame or a tree.

There are safety issues with climbing trees so finding a safe environment with climbing frames and nets is probably a wise decision.

Many towns now also have Leisure Centres with climbing walls. They are safe and an instructor will always be at hand. Kids are taught how to use ropes and to climb efficiently. This can be an interesting hobby for a child.

Burns Calories, builds muscle. Because the kid will be hanging for long periods muscle endurance and strength is dramatically improved along with mental endurance.

Self-esteem is often raised. Time will fly with this fun activity!

Chapter Six - House Hold Activities and Lifestyle changes that 'Trick' a Kid into burning Calories.

In addition to fun activities to help a fat kid lose weight conventional household activities can be incorporated in to a kids exercise regime.

Stand up!

Sounds simple but many people don't realise that standing rather than sitting burns Calories.

In fact, even if a kid does absolutely nothing all day except eat and lay in bed, about ten percent of their usual energy expenditure is still used to digest and store the nutrients in the food they eat. The brain alone uses around 350 Calories a day to operate, the Liver 550 Calories a day just to function before any physical activity enters the equation.

'…STANDING BURNS MORE CALORIES THAN SITTING.'

In order to stand, the body needs to remain stable and up-right. Core muscles in particular burn energy keeping a kid from falling over! It is admittedly an unconscious process but the core muscles along with the leg and back muscle continuously contract and relax to keep a human up-right.

Walk with the Phone

Today kids spend hours on their Phones, talking and text their friends, surfing the web and downloading applications.

If you encourage a Child to walk around the house when on the phone the calories burnt dramatically increase. It is a small change that can make a big difference.

Hide the Remote Control!

I think it has become universally accepted that kids need to spend less time in front of the TV and Video games.

Watching too much TV is associated with a sedentary lifestyle leading to increased weight and obesity so it is something that needs to be addressed.

It is difficult to regulate the exact time a kid is in front of a TV, or video game especially when they sometimes need to watch a programme for school or their parents just feel it is educational. So one solution to this is to try to break up the amount of sitting down that is accomplished.

'...HELP THEM RETAIN INFORMATION'.

Just having to get up to switch the channels might be good enough to get a kid moving.

Once they are out of their seat perhaps they could be encouraged to participate in some light activity between programs or adverts?

Just as stated previously, Hula Hooping between commercials can burn a great deal of fat and it helps get a kids brain oxygenated if they are watching an educational programme for school. Helping them to retain the information!

You could of course be really mean and make them stand whilst watching TV! Standing burns more calories than sitting and I bet the amount of TV watched will cut down if they have to stand!

Wash and/or Polishing the Car

Washing a car is quite low in intensity and to many kids it is enjoyable. It can easily become a Cardio activity if the pace is increased, challenging a kid to wash a car in a given time could give him or her a great workout.

Polishing a car uses much more muscle as it is required that a certain amount of force is applied especially in polishing off the residual. For this reason polishing a car is considered a muscle building activity. The main benefit is you get your car polished!

'…POLISHING BUILDS MORE MUSCLE.'

One way to 'trick' your kid into this activity on a regular basis is to allow them to wash the neighbours cars for money. A small money making enterprise where the kid not only gets some extra cash to spend but inadvertently loses weight! Just make sure they don't go to the store and spend their money on Candy!

Mowing the Lawn

Pushing a lawn mower takes a considerable amount of energy and muscular activity especially when turning the machine.

It is a great way to get a kid out into the fresh air and moving. Compliment them on a good job or challenge them to mow stripes on the lawn in order to engage them mentally in the task.

'...A GREAT WAY TO GET A KID OUT INTO THE FREASH AIR AND MOVING.'

We mentioned earlier about the language you use. Household activities are areas where this is very important. If you call an activity such as mowing the lawn or washing the car or even taking the trash out a *chore*, then that creates resistance. However much a kid enjoys an activity once it is labeled a chore it becomes one and it is less desirable. Many kids enjoy washing cars or mowing the lawn so become aware of how you label things.

References

Introduction.

*1 - Alison Jeffery, Peninsula Medical School of Exeter and Plymouth Universities, EarlyBird study, March 2004, earlbirddiabetestrust.org.
*2 - Dietary Fat Intake and the Risk of Depression: The SUN Project." - Almudena Sánchez-Villegas, Lisa Verberne, Jokin De Irala, Miguel Ruíz-Canela, Estefanía Toledo, Lluis Serra-Majem, Miguel Angel Martínez-González. *PLoS ONE*, 6(1): e16268; published online 26 Jan 2011.
DOI:10.1371/journal.pone.0016268
*3 - Physical Activity and Cancer Risk - The Cancer.Net Editorial Board, 6/2011.http://www.cancer.net/patient/All+About+Cancer/Risk+Factors+and+Prevention/Physical+Activity/Physical+Activity+and+Cancer+Risk

Chapter One.

*1 - *IASO/IOTF, http://www.iaso.org/iotf/ - international obesity taskforce.*
*2 - *(from the National Health and Nutrition Examination Survey (NHANES) http://www.cdc.gov/nchs/nhanes.htm & http://www.cdc.gov Centres for Disease Control and Prevention)*
*3 - Ogden CL, Carroll MD, Curtin LR, Lamb MM, Flegal KM. Prevalence of high body mass index in U.S. children and adolescents, 2007-2008. JAMA. 2010;303(3):242-249.
*4, 5 - Flegal KM, Carroll MD, Ogden CL, Curtin LR. Prevalence and trends in obesity among U.S. adults, 1999-2008. JAMA. 2010;303(3):235-241.
*6 - Centers for Disease Control and Prevention. National Diabetes Fact Sheet, 2007. http://www.cdc.gov/diabetes/pubs/pdf/ndfs_2007.pdf. Estimates projected to U.S. population in 2009.
*7 - Report in Academic Pediatrics by an obesity expert at Brenner Children's Hospital, part of Wake Forest University Baptist Medical Center. - Joseph A. Skelton, Stephen R. Cook, Peggy Auinger, Jonathan D. Klein, Sarah E. Barlow Prevalence and Trends of Severe Obesity Among US Children and Adolescents
Academic Pediatrics   2009 July
Department of Pediatrics, Wake Forest University School of Medicine, Winston-Salem, NC.
*8 - Dr. Giorgio Radetti, Department of Pediatrics, Regional Hospital, via L. Boehler 5, 39100 Bolzano, Italy.
http://jcem.endojournals.org/content/93/12/4749.full?sid=060d3fe5-7a8c-40fd-8504-396939995f8c.
*9 - Centers for Disease Control and Prevention. National Diabetes Fact Sheet,

2007. http://www.cdc.gov/diabetes/pubs/pdf/ndfs_2007.pdf.
*10 - Sleep problems in overweight children appear fairly common. Dr. Catherine L. Davis, MCG clinical health psychologist.& Dr. Amy R. Blanchard, pulmonologist and director of the MCG Georgia Sleep Center. Nov 2006 Obesity.
*11 - National Cancer Institute. Surveillance Epidemiology and End Results (SEER) Stat Fact Sheets: All Sites. http://seer.cancer.gov/statfacts/html/all.html.

Chapter Two.

*1 - Source: Institute of Medicine. Dietary Reference Intakes for Energy, Carbohydrate, Fiber, Fat, Fatty Acids, Cholesterol, Protein, and Amino Acids. Washington (DC): The National Academies Press; 2002.

*2 - Ogden CL, Carroll MD, Curtin LR, Lamb MM, Flegal KM. Prevalence of high body mass index in U.S. children and adolescents, 2007-2008. JAMA. 2010;303(3):242-249.

*3 - *UK Department of Health Estimated Average Requirements (EAR)*

*4 - Source: Institute of Medicine. Dietary Reference Intakes for Energy, Carbohydrate, Fiber, Fat, Fatty Acids, Cholesterol, Protein, and Amino Acids. Washington (DC): The National Academies Press; 2002.

*5, 8 –Halberg, F (1983). Chronobiology and nutrition. ***Contemporary Nutrition 9.***

*6 - Source: Institute of Medicine. Dietary Reference Intakes for Energy, Carbohydrate, Fiber, Fat, Fatty Acids, Cholesterol, Protein, and Amino Acids. Washington (DC): The National Academies Press; 2002.

*7 - Myers, RD and ML McCaleb. "Feeding: satiety signal from intestine triggers brain's noradrenergic mechanism." Science, Vol 209, Issue 4460, 1035-1037. http://www.sciencemag.org/cgi/content/abstract/209/4460/1035

*9 - *(Pollitt 1995 - Journal of the American Dietetic Association, Volume 95, Issue 10, Pages 1134-1139, October 1995 - Ernesto Pollitt PhD).*

*10, 11, 12 - *Nancy Clarke – sports nutrition guidebook, p62, breakfast is for champions.*

Chapter Three.

*1 - 'The colour red reduces snack food and soft drink intake' – by Oliver Genschow, Leonie Reutner, Michaela Wänke. University of Basel, Department of Social and Economic Psychology, Missionsstrasse 62A, 4055 Basel, Switzerland, University of Mannheim, Dept. of Consumer Psychology, Parkring 47, 68159 Mannheim, Germany. Published by The Journal Appetite**,** Available online 5 January 2012.

*2 - ***Family Matters****: Substance Abuse and the American Family - March 2005 - http://www.iowadec.net/uploads/380-family_matters_report.pdf.*

*3 - researcher Kerri N. Boutelle, PhD. She is an associate professor of pediatrics and psychiety at University of California-San Diego and Rady

Chapter Four.

*1 - Biddle, S. (1995) Exercise and psychological health. *Research Quarterly for Exercise and Sport* **66,** 292-297.

*2 - **Epidemiological evidence for the role of physical activity in reducing risk of type 2 diabetes and cardiovascular disease -** Shari S. Bassuk[1] and JoAnn E. Manson. Div. of Preventive Medicine, Brigham and Women's Hospital, 900 Commonwealth Ave., Boston, MA 02215.

*3 - Physical Activity and Cancer Risk - **This section has been reviewed and approved by the Cancer.Net Editorial Board, 6/2011.**
http://www.cancer.net/patient/All+About+Cancer/Risk+Factors+and+Prevention/Physical+Activity/Physical+Activity+and+Cancer+Risk.

*4 - **Study Shows Regular Exercise Benefits Prostate Cancer Survivors -** Article date: January 7, 2010, By: Rebecca Viksnins Snowden.

*5 - Physical activity and the risk of colon cancer among women: a prospective cohort study (united states). "Published online Feb. 17, 2006, in the *International Journal of Cancer*. First author: Brook A. Calton, University of California, San Francisco.

*6 - *Dietary Fat Intake and the Risk of Depression: The SUN Project." -* Almudena Sánchez-Villegas, Lisa Verberne, Jokin De Irala, Miguel Ruíz-Canela, Estefanía Toledo, Lluis Serra-Majem, Miguel Angel Martínez-González. *PLoS ONE*, 6(1): e16268; published online 26 Jan 2011.
DOI:10.1371/journal.pone.0016268.

*7 - http://www.nhs.uk/Livewell/fitness/Pages/physical-activity-guidelines-for-children.aspx

*8, Borg G.A. Psychophysical bases of perceived exertion. *Medicine and Science in Sports and Exercise*. 1982; 14:377-381. Department of Clinical Sciences, The University of Chester, Cheshire, UK.

*9 - **The Nutrition Source - The Borg Scale of Perceived Exertion.**
http://www.hsph.harvard.edu/nutritionsource/staying-active/borg-scale/.

Chapter Five.

*1 - http://www.nhs.uk

Copyright and Disclaimer

COPYRIGHT AND TRADEMARK NOTICES
Copyright © 2012 Stephen Mycoe (the "Author"). All Rights Reserved.

No part of this Book may be reproduced or transmitted in any form or by any means, electronic or mechanical, including photocopying, recording, or by an information storage and retrieval system (except by a reviewer who may quote brief passages in a review to be printed in a magazine, newspaper, blog, or website on the condition that the quote is fully referenced to the original work) without permission in writing from the Author.

LIMITS OF LIABILITY & DISCLAIMERS OF WARRANTIES
This Book is a general educational health-related information product.

As an express condition to reading this Book, you understand and agree to the following terms.

The Book's content is not a substitute for direct, personal, professional medical and/or nutritional care and diagnosis. None of the exercises and/or activities or treatments (including products and services) mentioned in this Book should be performed or otherwise used without advice from your physician, health care provider or Nutritionist, by yourself or any other persons associated with the reader.

The materials in this Book are provided "as is" and without warranties of any kind either expressed or implied. The Author disclaims all warranties, expressed or implied, including, but not limited to, implied warranties of merchantability, health and fitness for a particular purpose.

The Author does not warrant or make any representations regarding the use or the results of the use of the materials in this

Book in terms of their correctness, accuracy, reliability, or otherwise. Applicable law may not allow the exclusion of implied warranties, so the above exclusion may not apply to you. Under no circumstances, including, but not limited to, negligence, shall the Author be liable for any special or consequential damages that result from the use of, or the inability to use this Book.

You agree to hold the Author of this Book, the Author's owners, agents, affiliates, and employees harmless from any and all liability for all claims for damages due to injuries, including lawyer fees and costs, incurred by you or caused to third parties by you, arising out of the products, services, and activities discussed in this Book.

Facts and information are believed to be accurate at the time they were placed in this Book. All data provided in this Book is to be used for information purposes only. The information contained within is not intended to provide specific physical or mental health advice, or any other advice whatsoever, for any individual or company and should not be relied upon in that regard. The services described are only offered in jurisdictions where they may be legally offered. Information provided is not all-inclusive, and is limited to information that is made available and such information should not be relied upon as all-inclusive or accurate.

ABOUT THE AUTHOR

About Steve

Author and Sports Hypnotist Steve has over a decade of experience in Sports Hypnosis and Body Conditioning. A former University boxer and dedicated athlete Steve has an inside knowledge of performance enhancement second to none. He is qualified by the 'British Weight Lifters Association' to instruct, a certified Boxing Instructor and has qualifications in Counseling.

Steve's first book **'Unlimited Sports Success** – *the Power of Hypnosis*' was published in 2001 and documents his work with athletes. He has published over sixty books and CD's. Steve's books and best selling Sports Hypnosis CD's have helped to inspire, develop and motivate athletes worldwide.

Other health related books by Steve include; **'How to Skip Like a Boxer** – *to Lose Weight, Tone-Up, Get Fit and feel Great!*' and **'How to Hula Hoop** – *to Lose Weight and Feel like a Kid Again!*' all available on Amazon and Kindle.

For more information visit his website
www.SportsHypnosis.co.uk

Printed in Great Britain
by Amazon.co.uk, Ltd.,
Marston Gate.